I0408603

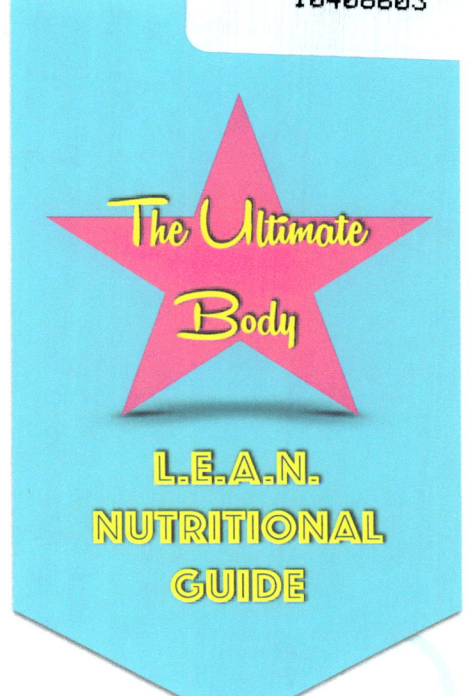

The Ultimate Body

L.E.A.N. NUTRITIONAL GUIDE

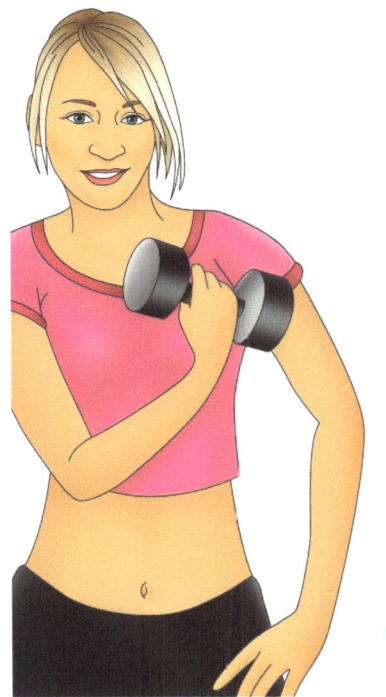

Lesley Morrison Fitness
www.lmfitness.info

PRODUCT DISCLAIMER

All of the information and instructions contained within the booklet have been produced and written by Lesley Morrison of LM Fitness.

The contents within this Ultimate Body L.E.A.N Nutrition Guide, has been developed and designed to assist in the improvements of general health, fitness and physique in line with current health organisation guidelines.

The meals contained within this guide have not been designed or tailored for one specific individual, nor have they been created with any medical conditions or health problems in mind other than weight related issues. It is recommended that you seek the advice of your medical professional prior to embarking on any new nutritional or activity plan in order to ascertain
its suitability to your particular health & fitness requirements.

The booklet has been written as an educational source of information and assistance for those participants wishing to achieve fitness and physique changes, however Lesley Morrison & LM Fitness are not, and cannot be held responsible, nor liable for any misuse, overuse or injury that may be incurred during a participants practise of the guide.

The guidelines set within this guide, although set to over a duration, make no indication that participants will achieve a total body transformation within this timespan. All participants commence their journey at different ages, sizes, paths and abilities. This programme can be repeated and/or continued if participants follow it accordingly.

The information within this booklet have been collated from personal experiences by Lesley Morrison of LM Fitness, with training clients. Accordingly the information within this booklet is copyright 2012 ©LM Fitness.

The contents of this guide should not be reproduced, manually, electronically, written or otherwise. It may not be sold by any other means that Lesley Morrison, LM Fitness, UK

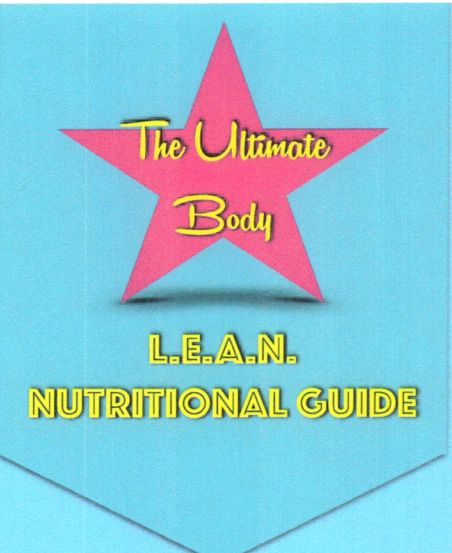

About Your Trainer

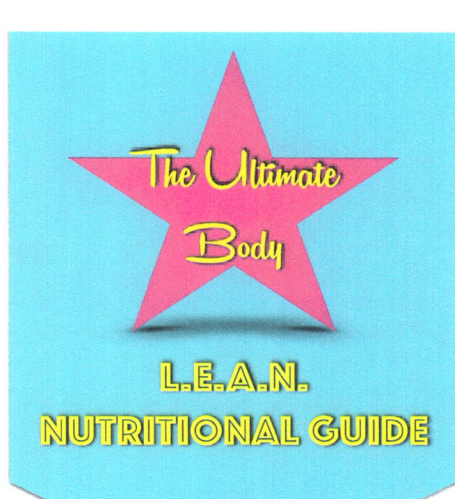

Lesley Morrison

Owner & Trainer
LM Fitness

I began my transformation to the Fitness Industry in 2007, after many years of being a happy "Gym Bunny". Turning one of my passions into a career seemed the logical thing to do. Turned out it was one of the best things I ever did!

At the age of 27, I went from being a desk jockey to a Personal Trainer, and already had a great job lined up with a national gym chain. I put my head down and learnt everything I could from the guys & girls in the gym. And soon after completing my Diploma in Fitness & Nutrition with Future Fit Training, and spending a very happy few years working within the gym, I made the bold decision to take my career freelance.

In 2011, I completed my GP Referral Consultation and Pre & Post Natal Diplomas, and expanded my knowledge and client base. Becoming a specialist trainer.

In 2012, I had already a massed over 300 clients, and was running several very successful bootcamps and ladies only fitness classes.

In 2013, I launched my online Clean Living Nutrition Programme, which caught the attention of people as far afield as the USA, India & Russia.

In 2014, I launched an online training programme, which has now been superseded with this and many other Fitness Guides, all available via the Website. I also successfully published three Ebooks with Amazon.

To this day, in 2015, I still have many of my original clients, whose goals keep evolving as they do, the fitness classes are still growing and I am always looking for new innovative ways to help as many people I can realise their true potential, without costing the earth.

I hope that you enjoy the guide, and I wish the very best of luck in achieving as much from what I tell you over the pages, as many people before you have.

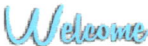

Welcome

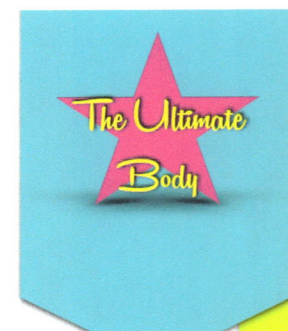

Welcome to the L.E.A.N. Nutrition Guide, part of the Ultimate Body Workout.

Firstly, thank you so much for purchasing the guide, and I hope that you achieve every success with this guide as not only I have, but many of my clients before you.

The Guide is set out in to easy to follow plans, with recipes, and alternatives included.

Healthy eating is essential for everyone, and not just from a weight loss perspective, but from a health and well being view as well.

This Guide will help you to make educated choices about the foods you eat, when you eat them and also how you prepare them. It should not be viewed as a diet, but as a lifestyle alteration.

L.E.A.N., in short refers to Lifestyle, Exercise and Nutrition, so we will cover aspects of all three in this guide. However, for a more in-depth guide to exercise and activity, you should download the Ultimate Body 12 Week Workout Guide.

The two guides have been created to work side by side and hand in hand to help you achieve what you want. The Ultimate Body, does not refer to a size, a weight or a specific body type. It is individual to you. Your Ultimate Body is the one that you are happy in. When you look in the mirror, you feel satisfied with the reflection looking back. Confident, Sexy, Attractive.

Although we do monitor progression with the guides, we do not state a timeframe. Weight loss, Transformations and physique improvements take time, and we all start our journeys at different stages.

And what is more, these changes that we all desire, are the result of not one action, but many. Nutrition, Lifestyle and Activity are key in these changes, and one without the other will not yield the results as much as all combined.

©LM Fitness 2015

Before you begin your journey with the guide, take some time to read through the whole booklet. If you print the book, scribble notes where you need to, this guide is yours and yours only, and your journey will be as individual as you.

Look through the recipes and meal plans, and start compiling your weekly shopping list to suit your plans.

Our health is important to us, and it starts within. Cleansing our bodies from the inside out will make a huge impact on your mental well being, as well as your physical.

More energy, clearer thinking, greater alertness, healthier skin, hair, nails and so much more.

Fail to plan, and you are planning to fail.

With this guide, you should plan to succeed, like so many others have. Step out of your routines, move away from the unhealthy snacks and start giving your body the fuel and nutrients it needs to thrive.

Remember to track your progress using photographic evidence. There is a page towards the back of this manual to explain how to take your photos and when.

Have an amazing time working through the guide, and I wish you every success.

What is Healthy Nutrition

Nutrition can be a minefield of confusion for many people. So over the next few pages, I am going to try and help you understand the fundamentals of this topic.

As already mentioned, this guide should be used a lifestyle alteration rather than a diet. A diet implies that there is a expiration date, at which time normal habits can resume. The result being that although you may have lost the weight you wanted, if your habits haven't changed, you will end up eventually over time returning back to your starting point.
And that is the last thing we want.

We want to lose weight in the hope that it is exactly that…. Lost, and not to be found again!
This is why I say it is a lifestyle alteration, and as with most things, it takes time to get it right.

Your "diet" should supply you with adequate calories to fuel your bodies essential day to day organ functions, this includes imperative actions such as your breathing, your heart beating, your brain function and everything else your body does involuntarily on a daily basis!

Calories are something that most people will refer to as the thing we need to reduce in order to lose weight. But do you understand Calories? If not, then how do you know what is required.

Although we are not "*calorie counting*" throughout this guide, for your information, I am going to explain (in brief) what calories are.

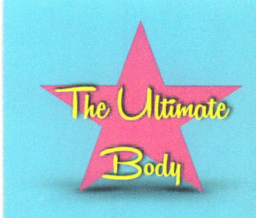

WHAT ARE CALORIES?

Calories are not a protein, fat or carbohydrate, nor are they a vitamin or mineral. A Calorie is a simple measurement of energy. Without getting too technical, 1 calorie is the amount of energy required to increase the temperature of 1 gram of water by 1 degree.

We use calories to recognise which foods contain what amount of energy. But it's easy to be confused by calories, as there is such as thing as an "empty" calorie.

These "Empty" calories tend to be in sweets, highly processed foods & alcohol. Empty calories have no nutritional value to our bodies. So it is important to try and reduce the amount of these we consume. Despite them having no nutritional benefit, they will still add to your calories consumption every day.

Foods that are high in calorie content are not necessarily bad for us either.

As I've already mentioned, we are not calorie counting throughout this guide, so I am not going to go into too much depth on what a calorie is, however, it is important to ensure that we are not eating too many, nor too few, as both ends of the spectrum can have a negative effect on our health.

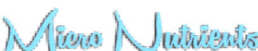

Micro Nutrients

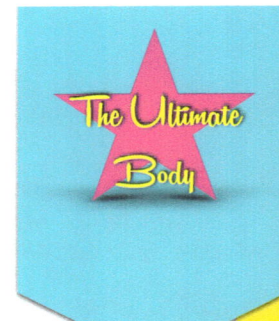

Within our "diets" we need micronutrients and macronutrients. But, what are these? It is important to understand what your body needs in order to supply the right kind of fuel.

To start with lets take a look at Micronutrients.

Micronutrients are required in small amounts, but despite this they are essential for good health. Deficiencies in micronutrients can lead to some serious health implications.

(There is quite a long list of these essential Micro nutrients on the following page for you.)

Micronutrients include such dietary minerals like zinc and iodine, both of which are necessary for the healthy function of all of your bodies systems, from the growth and health of your bones to the functionality of your brain.

In short, Micronutrients are what we call Vitamins & Minerals, and they all play a vital role in your bodies health and well being.

Achieving the right amount of these Micronutrients isn't difficult when eating a healthy and balanced, nutritious diet.

Colour is key here, as colours can represent the various mineral and vitamin content. The more colour the better!

A deficiency in micronutrients can lead to some unfavourable health problems. The World Health Organisation suggests that micronutrient deficiency presents a huge threat to the health of the worlds population. Some more common deficiencies include Iodine, vitamin A and Iron.

As the population moves to more convenient, quick, processed meals and foods, the nutritional value of the food is often compromised through all of the processing.

This guide will help you to increase your Micronutrient intake to a healthy level and maintain it.

Check out all of the MicroNutrients on the following page.

Micro Nutrients

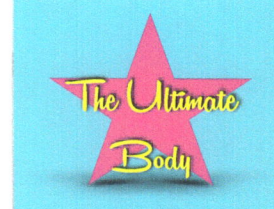

VITAMINS
★ Vitamin C
★ Vitamin B3 (Niacin)
★ Vitamin B5 (Pantothenate)
★ Vitamin B1 (Thiamine)
★ Vitamin B2 (Riboflavin)
★ Vitamin B6 (Pyridoxine)
★ Vitamin B12 (Cyanocobalamin)
★ Folic Acid
★ Biotin
★ Beta-Carotene
★ Vitamin D3
★ Vitamin E (d-alpha-Tocopherol)

MINERALS
★ Magnesium
★ Calcium
★ Potassium
★ Phosphorus

TRACE ELEMENTS
★ Zinc
★ Magnesium
★ Copper
★ Selenium
★ Chromium
★ Molybdenum

AMINO ACIDS
★ Taurine
★ L-Lysine
★ L-Proline
★ L-Arginine
★ L-Carnitine
★ L-Cysteine

Macro Nutrients

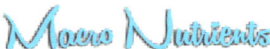

As the name suggest, Macronutrients are needed in larger quantities than micronutrients. There are three macronutrients in nutrition, and they are carbohydrates, lipids (fats), and proteins.

What are Macronutrients?

Macronutrients are the dominant provider of energy that the body needs for growth and bodily functions. These are our main providers of calories.

The amount of calories per macronutrient is calculated by the weight. For example:
- In carbohydrates, there are 4 calories per gram
- In proteins, there are 4 calories per gram
- And in lipids (fats), there are 9 calories per gram

We need carbohydrates in the largest quantities. They are easily metabolised (broken down) and are used as the body's main source of energy. There are two types of carbohydrates, simple and complex.
Simple Carbs are sugar, whereas complex carbs are predominantly starchy foods. The difference really comes down to how quickly they burn off in the body. Simple carbs (sugars) burn off very quickly and give a quick energy boost, and complex carbs are more slow releasing and sustain your energy levels over a longer period.

Fibre is also an indigestible form of Carbohydrate. Our bodies cannot break down these Fibre Carbohydrates and they pass through our digestive system whole, taking other waste products with them.
Reducing your fibre intake can cause some digestive health implications, such as constipation & haemorrhoids.

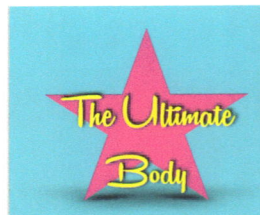

Protein is also vital for the reconstruction, maintenance and repair of most cells within the body. Protein also regulates & maintains the main bodily functions.
The enzymes that are used for immunity & digestion are also made of proteins, and all of the essential hormones used by the body all require protein.
When carbohydrates run low, protein can also be used a form of energy.

The body breaks proteins down into what is called Amino-Acids. There are over 500 of these so I shall not list them all. But 21 of them are necessary for life, 9 of which are "essential" as the body cannot produce them, so they must be consumed in foods or supplements.

Finally you have lipids (fats), of which there is saturated and unsaturated. Fat is probably what people know the most about, due to the extensive media that has surrounded the intake of fat, and which is good and which is bad.
We need fat within our diets for things like the maintenance of cell membranes. Lipids are also a high-density energy source and help us to absorb fat soluble vitamins.

It would not be wise to completely cut out any one group of foods, as they all play their role in our function.

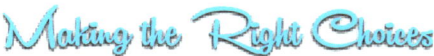

Making the Right Choices

So, now we know what Micro & Macro Nutrients are, we can start to look at foods and make more educated choices on what we should be eating.

Understanding what is in your food, will help you to understand what you are putting in to, not only your bodies, but your families as well.

Remember what I said earlier, that colour is key?
You should eat the rainbow.

The NHS, here in the UK recommend five portions of fruit and/or vegetables per day, but this has recently been argued by other organisations and health professionals. In studies they found that ten portions was significantly better for our health than the original five. They also found in this study that vegetables were greater in nutrients and health benefits than fruit. The jury is still out on the 10-a-day theory, but I personally agree that Vegetables are much better than fruit.

The main point here, is that you should be eating plenty of healthy, colourful fruit & vegetables EVERY day. And that will be reflected during this guide.

In addition, you will need to be drinking at least 2 litres of water daily. Water is essential to our bodies, and a well hydrated body will perform & feel much better. Being well hydrated not only helps you to function, but it can help to improve headaches, skin problems, dry hair & nails and many other issues that modern day life throws at us.

Understanding Nutrition

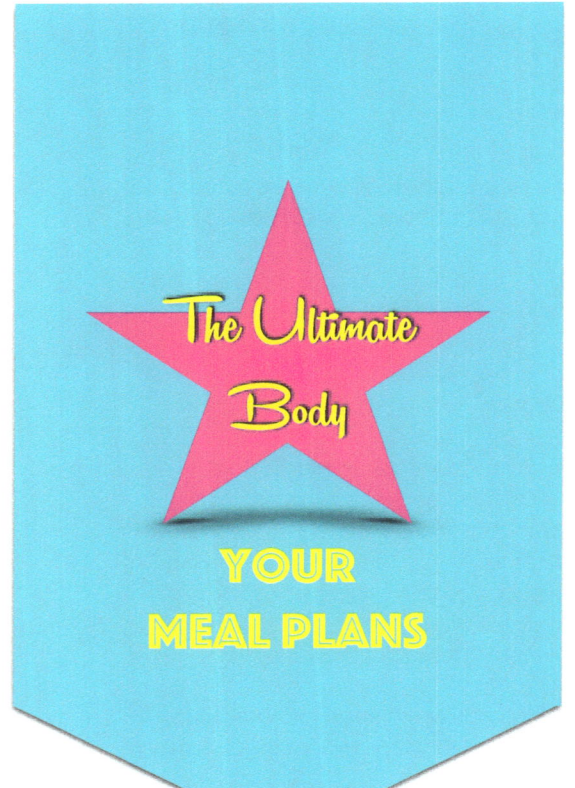

The Ultimate
Body

YOUR
MEAL PLANS

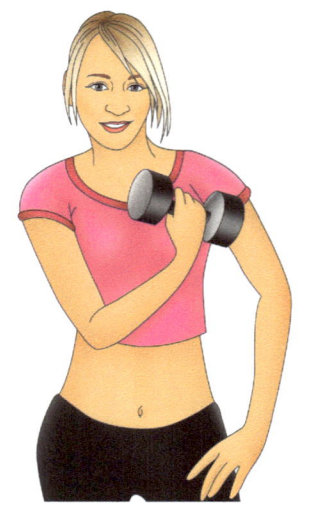

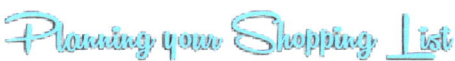

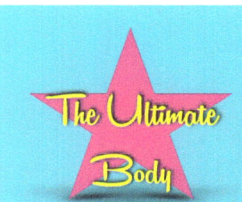

Before you start your journey with this guide, there are a few things you may need to go and get in order to be prepared. And being prepared is KEY!

So I have set out a few "go gets" for you here.

* Protein Powder
* B.C.A.A.'s
* MultiVitamin
* Omega 3, 6 & 9 Capsules
* Tupperware Tubs

This may sound like a lot to start with, however, check out the daily meal plans to see when and where each should be used. Also, if you are a vegetarian, check that the items are suitable, as not all capsules and proteins are vegetarian/vegan friendly.

Protein Powder is great for aiding muscle recovery after a workout, and repairing the muscle fibres that you have damaged during a the exercise. It is the 24 hours DOMS that indicate how much you have torn your muscle fibres, and if you have ever experienced DOMS you will know it can be quite unpleasant if you have over stepped the mark with your effort levels, or if you are returning to exercise after a long period of inactivity.

B.C.A.A's are Branch Chain Amino Acids and are essential for the body. As the body cannot make these Amino Acids from other cells, it is always worth considering taking a capsules to ensure your body receives them. Furthermore, B.C.A.A's can aid peak functionality of the body. If you have something missing from your system, how can you expect to function optimally?

MultiVitamins are always useful, again to ensure that the body has all of the essential micronutrients that it requires for optimal function.

The best example I can give for both B.C.A.A''s & MultiVitamins, is this:

Imagine a chain with a broken link, the chain can't possible function to its best ability. The links connecting to the damaged one, as well as the damaged link itself, will all be under additional stress to hold the chain together. Eventually the chain will break and it can no longer be used. Now, imagine our body and all its cells working to achieve optimal performance, but there is something missing. Suddenly the "chain" is under stress and failing to do what it needs to do. Completing that chain by adding the Essential Amino Acids & MicroNutrients, will restore the strength of the chain and allow the body to return to peak operation.

Finally, **Omega 3, 6 & 9**. Again, these Fatty Acids, are important for optimal health. Omega 3 & 6 are essential as the body cannot produce them on its own. They come with added benefits, like anti-inflammatory properties that enhance joint health & healing, they may also help to prevent certain diseases.
Studies have shown that taking "fish oil" at the start of your day can help to break down fatty deposits and aid you in weight loss. So this is why I include them.

All of the above are "aids", not answers! You will still need to eat well and incorporate activity to achieve results!

Day One

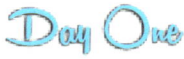

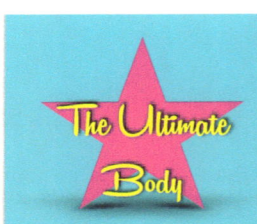

When starting any new lifestyle choice, you need to plan. Failing to do so is like planning to fail. Make sure that you have read through all of this weeks food choices, purchased everything you need for the week ahead and planned what you are eating and when. If you know about a day out or an event, plan your meals and where you are eating for this day, and try to avoid any unhealthy

Meal One:

★ 1/2 a cup of porridge oats, prepared in water, mix 1/2 scoop of Protein powder into the mix, & serve with 8-12 blueberries & 1/3 of a Banana sliced
  - ★ Glass of Water
  - ★ BCAA
  - ★ MultiVitamin
  - ★ Omega 3, 6 & 9 Capsule
★ 1 Cup of Green Tea & Lemon, no added milk or sugar

Meal Two:

★ 1/2 a cup of plain Almond Nuts

Meal Three:

★ 1 Grilled Chicken Breast, 1/2 Avocado sliced, 1/2 a cup of raw Green Beans (wash first)
  - ★ Serve with 1 teaspoon of Mayonnaise or Houmous
  - ★ Glass of Water
★ 1 Cup of Green Tea with Lemon, no added milk or sugar

Meal Four:

★ 1 Cup of Carrot Sticks, served with Houmous

Meal Five:

★ 1 Salmon Fillet, 1 Cup of Mixed Green Vegetables, 2 Asparagus stalks
  - ★ Glass of Water

Meal Six:

★ 1/2 Banana or 1/2 a Cup of Unsalted Nuts (cashews, almonds, brazil)
  - ★ Glass of Water

Throughout the day you should consume AT LEAST 2 litres of water, so drink frequently. Hydration is essential for remaining healthy and weight loss.

You should also aim to get 7-8 hours sleep per night for optimal health, recovery and results.

Day Two

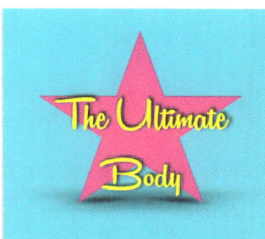

Health and Fitness is not a luxury, but a necessity. The body asks for fluid in the same way that it asks for food, that grumble in your stomach. Before you reach for nibbles, reach for water. If tap water isn't something you enjoy, try boiling it and adding a slice of lemon to it, for a refreshing citrus flavour.

Remember though, if your tummy is grumbling, you may have waited too long, eat at regular intervals. I recommend, breakfast between 6 & 7.30, a snack around 10.30, Lunch between 12 and 1.30pm, another snack at about 3pm, dinner between 6pm and 7.30 and your final snack around 8.30-9pm.

Meal One:

★ 1 slice of Rye Bread (toasted), with 2 scrambled or poached eggs.
- ★ Glass of Water
- ★ BCAA
- ★ MultiVitamin
- ★ Omega 3, 6 & 9 Capsule

★ 1 Cup of Green Tea & Lemon, no added milk or sugar

Meal Two:

★ 1 Scoop of Protein powder, prepared with water (shake/stir well)

Meal Three:

★ 1 tin of Tuna, with Mixed green salad and 6 carrot sticks
- ★ Serve with 1 teaspoon of Mayonnaise or Humous
- ★ Glass of Water

★ 1 Cup of Green Tea with Lemon, no added milk or sugar

Meal Four:

★ Two tbsp of Natural Greek Yoghurt, with a small handful of Berries, 1 small sprinkle of cinnamon

Meal Five:

★ 1 Lean Beef burger (grilled), 2 cups of steamed mixed vegetables, 1 tsp of homemade salsa
- ★ Glass of Water

Meal Six:

★ 1 cup of Carrot sticks or Celery with 1 tsp of Mayonnaise
- ★ Glass of Water

Week One

Day Three

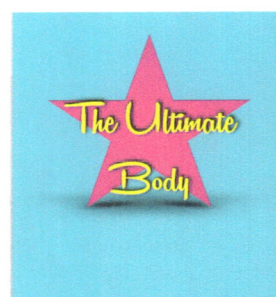

Being active will boost your results and energy. If you work in a sedentary environment, sitting behind a desk or driving a lot, try and get out of your seat at least once an hour and move. Even if this is just standing up behind your desk, it helps to increase your energy expenditure. You should aim for at least 3 dedicated exercise sessions per week, for at least 45-60minutes each.

Meal One:
★ 1 slice of Sunflower Rye Bread (toasted), 2 sardines (in water), 1 egg boiled & sliced
  - ★ Glass of Water
  - ★ BCAA
  - ★ MultiVitamin
  - ★ Omega 3, 6 & 9 Capsule
★ 1 Cup of Green Tea & Lemon, no added milk or sugar

Meal Two:
★ 2 tbsp of Natural Nut Butter or Organic Peanut Butter

Meal Three:
★ 1/2 Grilled Turkey Breast, 2 Asparagus stalks, 1/2 a Cup of Carrot Sticks
  - ★ Serve with 1 teaspoon of Houmous
  - ★ Glass of Water
★ 1 Cup of Green Tea with Lemon, no added milk or sugar

Meal Four:
★ 1 Apple, 5 or 6 Plain Almond Nuts OR 3-4 Plain Macadamia Nuts

Meal Five:
★ 1 Fillet of Smoked Mackerel (plain), Mixed Salad (lettuce, tomato, cucumber, avocado),
  - ★ Serve with a squeeze of Lemon Juice and a small tsp of Mayonnaise or Home made Salsa
  - ★ Glass of Water

Meal Six:
★ 1 Scoop of Protein Powder with Water or Almond Milk

Week One

Day Four

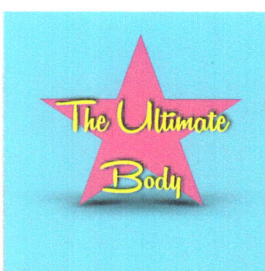

Grazing throughout the day, eating smaller meals more often with boost your metabolism and aid weight control or weight loss. You should not avoid any one group of MacroNutrients in any "diet". Moderation and serving sizes are key to results and energy levels. You should not feel tired nor lethargic when eating a balanced & healthy diet.

Meal One:
★ 1/2 a Cup of Porridge Oats (cooked in water), 3 chopped Strawberries, 1/2 a scoop of Protein Powder
    ★ Glass of Water
    ★ BCAA
    ★ MultiVitamin
    ★ Omega 3, 6 & 9 Capsule
★ 1 Cup of Green Tea & Lemon, no added milk or sugar

Meal Two:
★ 1 tbsp of Cottage Cheese, 1 Dark Rye Crispbread

Meal Three:
★ 2 Boiled eggs, sliced, 1 Asparagus stalk (cooked & cold)
    ★ Serve with 1 teaspoon of Houmous or Salad Cream
    ★ Glass of Water
★ 1 Cup of Green Tea with Lemon, no added milk or sugar

Meal Four:
★ 1/2 of a Banana & 5-6 Blueberries

Meal Five:
★ 1 Small Lean Frying Steak, 1 cup of Mixed Green Vegetables, 1/4 of an Avocado sliced
    ★ Serve with a small tsp of Mustard or Home made Salsa
    ★ Glass of Water

Meal Six:
★ 2 tbsp Natural Greek Yoghurt, 1 small sprinkle of cinnamon, 3 small grates of Dark Chocolate (80% cocoa or higher)

Remember to drink plenty of water, at least 2 litres per day. Try & reduce your intake of coffee and tea.

Week One

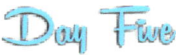

Day Five

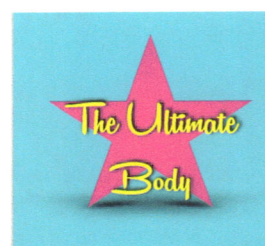

Tea & Coffee act as diuretics, meaning that they make you urinate more frequently. This can have a negative effect on your healthy diet, as the action of a diuretic can also purge your digestive system of healthy vitamins and minerals that the body may need to absorb. Too keep an optimal amount of nutrients in the body, try to reduce your intake of coffee and tea.

Meal One:

★ 2 Egg Omelette, with 1/2 cup of chopped green peppers and 1/4 cup of grated low fat cheese
  ★ Glass of Water
  ★ BCAA
  ★ MultiVitamin
  ★ Omega 3, 6 & 9 Capsule
★ 1 Cup of Green Tea & Lemon, no added milk or sugar

Meal Two:

★ 1/2 a Banana, sliced

Meal Three:

★ 1/2 a Sliced Chicken Breast, with a small amount of Lettuce, 1/4 of a raw courgette sliced
  ★ Serve with 1 teaspoon of Salsa
  ★ Glass of Water
★ 1 Cup of Green Tea with Lemon, no added milk or sugar

Meal Four:

★ 2 tbsp of Natural Greek Yoghurt, 1/2 scoop of Protein Powder and 2 sliced Strawberries

Meal Five:

★ 1 Swordfish Loin (grilled), Serve with 2 Grilled Cherry Tomatoes & 1 cup of Kale (steamed)
  ★ Serve with a small squeeze of Lemon juice
  ★ Glass of Water

Meal Six:

★ 2 tbsp Natural Greek Yoghurt, 1 small sprinkle of cinnamon, 3 small grates of Dark Chocolate (80% cocoa or higher)

Day Six

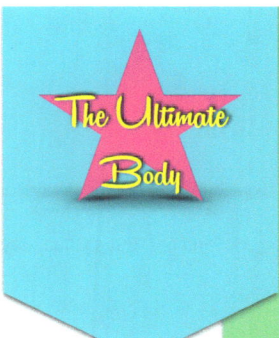

Having protein within our breakfast can sustain energy for longer, as it is slower burning that some traditional carbohydrate cereal breakfast, not to mention, there is generally a great amount of added sugar in cereal. Avoiding highly processed foods will give you clean energy throughout the day. Hence the phrase "Clean Diet".

Meal One:
★ 1/2 a Cup of Porridge Oat (cooked in water), 3-4 blackberries/raspberries, 1/2 scoop Protein Powder
  - ★ Glass of Water
  - ★ BCAA
  - ★ MultiVitamin
  - ★ Omega 3, 6 & 9 Capsule
★ 1 Cup of Green Tea & Lemon, no added milk or sugar

Meal Two:
★ 1/2 Cup of Plain Almond or Brazil Nuts

Meal Three:
★ 2 small slices of Smoked Salmon, with Dark Rye Crisp Bread and 1 tbsp of low fat Cream Cheese
  - ★ Glass of Water
★ 1 Cup of Green Tea with Lemon, no added milk or sugar

Meal Four:
★ 1/2 Cup of Carrot sticks with 1 tsp of houmous

Meal Five:
★ 2 Cups of Lean Mince Beef, with home made tomato sauce, served with a 1 & 1/2 cups of Wholemeal Pasta
  - ★ Glass of Water

Meal Six:
★ 8-12 Blueberries

Week One

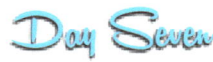

Day Seven

Your seventh day is a treat day, NOT A CHEAT DAY! The difference here is that on a treat day, you can chose one meal to have something a little naughty (in moderation). But a Cheat day is when all meals can be naughty... Do not get the

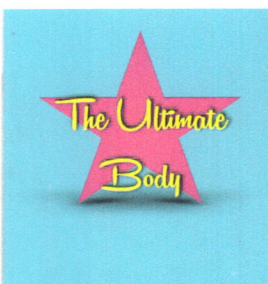

Meal One:
★ 2 Scrambled Eggs, on Rye Bread Toasted. Served with 1 sprig of Parsley and a small sprinkle   of salt &/or pepper
  - ★ Glass of Water
  - ★ BCAA
  - ★ MultiVitamin
  - ★ Omega 3, 6 & 9 Capsule
★ 1 Cup of Green Tea & Lemon, no added milk or sugar

Meal Two:
★ 1/2 Banana chopped/sliced

Meal Three:
★ 1 Small Grilled Chicken Breast, served with Mixed Green Vegetables
  - ★ Glass of Water
★ 1 Cup of Green Tea with Lemon, no added milk or sugar

Meal Four:
★ 1 Tbsp of Natural Greek Yoghurt with 3-6 Berries

Meal Five:
★ 4 Sliced of Roast Beef with mixed Vegetables and home made Gravy
  - ★ Glass of Water

Meal Six:
★ 1 Small portion of a treat of your choice. make sure your portion is sensible.

Week One Review

Now you have completed Week One of the Guide, you should be starting to feel more energy building in your body. You may feel less lethargic, and be noticing simple things like your eyes looking brighter.

You should also have experienced some inch or weight loss.

Well done to you for sticking to the plan.

Before we move on to week two, let's have a quick recap on what you should have done already!

- ★ Increased your water intake to 2litres per day
- ★ Decreased your intake of Tea & Coffee
- ★ Started preparing your meals & snacks
- ★ Taken your First "before" photo to track progress
- ★ Introduced a lot more colour into your diet

Your actions over the next few weeks will start to build the foundations of a habitual lifestyle alteration. All of which will be essential to your success using this plan, and beyond.

The Ultimate Body

IF YOU FAIL TO PLAN, YOU PLAN TO FAIL.

Week Two - Day One

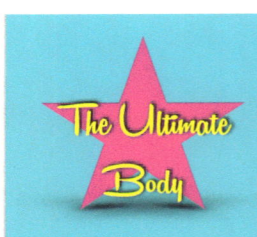

The first week of any new plan is always the hardest, and now you have got that out of the way, we can move on to week two. Our pattern of eating will remain unchanged, as we are forming healthy new habits. It can take up to 21 days to settle into a new routine, so make sure you maintain your focus and

Meal One:
★ 2 Sardines on Rye Bread Toasted, with 1 poached egg.
   - ★ Glass of Water
   - ★ BCAA
   - ★ MultiVitamin
   - ★ Omega 3, 6 & 9 Capsule
★ 1 Cup of Green Tea & Lemon, no added milk or sugar

Meal Two:
★ 1/4 of a Mango Diced

Meal Three:
★ 3 slices of Cooked Ham/Gammon, served with mixed Green vegetables
   - ★ Serve with 1 tsp of Mayonnaise
   - ★ Glass of Water
★ 1 Cup of Green Tea with Lemon, no added milk or sugar

Meal Four:
★ 1/2 a Cup of unsalted Macadamia Nuts

Meal Five:
★ 1/4 of a Home Made Quiche, Served with Mixed Salad (lettuce, rocket, 2 cherry tomatoes, 1/4 Courgette sliced.
   - ★ Glass of Water

Meal Six:
★ 2 tbsp of Natural Greek Yoghurt, with 1 small pinch of cinnamon and 3-5 berries.

Week Two

Week Two - Day Two

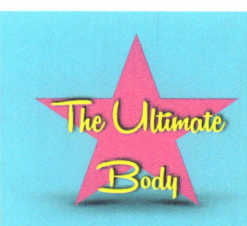

Every day is a new day, and a new day brings new exciting opportunities. With every day that passes whilst you enjoy the meals provided in this guide, your body is getting healthier, stronger and becoming much better at dealing with obstacles. Your body will do what ever your mind tells it too, and today we tell it to make smoothies!

Meal One:

★ 1/4 Mango, 6 Blueberries and 1/2 a Banana, mixed with 1 class of ice in a blender until smooth
  - ★ BCAA
  - ★ MultiVitamin
  - ★ Omega 3, 6 & 9 Capsule
★ 1 Cup of Green Tea & Lemon, no added milk or sugar

Meal Two:

★ 1 Tbsp Cottage Cheese on 1 Dark Rye Crispbread

Meal Three:

★ 1 tin of Tuna (in water) with 2 Asparagus stalks and mixed green Vegetables/Salad
  - ★ Serve with 1 tsp of Mayonnaise
  - ★ Glass of Water
★ 1 Cup of Green Tea with Lemon, no added milk or sugar

Meal Four:

★ 1/2 a Cup of Carrot Sticks

Meal Five:

★ 1 Grilled Chicken Breast, with 1/2 an Avocado, 1/2 a cup of Broccoli, 1/2 a cup of Spinach & 2 grilled cherry tomatoes.
  - ★ Glass of Water

Meal Six:

★ 2 tbsp Organic Peanut Butter

Week Two - Day Three

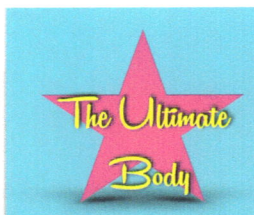

Preparing your meals and placing them in a tupperware tub in the fridge or freezer, is a great way to save time cooking every night. If you know you are due to be late home one evening, make your meals the day before and put them away ready to grab and go when you get in.

Meal One:
★ 1/2 a Cup of Porridge Oats (cooked in water), serve with 1/2 a Banana chopped and mix in 1/2 a scoop of Protein powder
  - ★ Glass of Water
  - ★ BCAA
  - ★ MultiVitamin
  - ★ Omega 3, 6 & 9 Capsule
★ 1 Cup of Green Tea & Lemon, no added milk or sugar

Meal Two:
★ 2 boiled eggs sliced

Meal Three:
★ Home Made Vegetable Soup
  - ★ Glass of Water
★ 1 Cup of Green Tea with Lemon, no added milk or sugar

Meal Four:
★ 1 Apple

Meal Five:
★ 1 Salmon fillet, served with 3 boiled New Potatoes, 1/2 a cup of Kale and 1/2 a cup of Baby Carrots
  - ★ Glass of Water

Meal Six:
★ 1/4 of a cup of Unsalted Brazil nuts

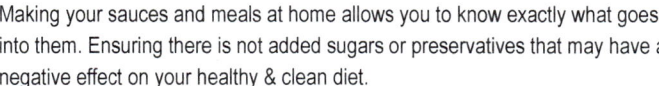

Week Two - Day Four

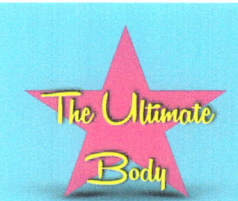

Making your sauces and meals at home allows you to know exactly what goes into them. Ensuring there is not added sugars or preservatives that may have a negative effect on your healthy & clean diet.

Meal One:

★ 1 slice of Sunflower Rye Bread (toasted), 2 sardines (in water), 1 egg boiled & sliced
  ★ Glass of Water
  ★ BCAA
  ★ MultiVitamin
  ★ Omega 3, 6 & 9 Capsule
★ 1 Cup of Green Tea & Lemon, no added milk or sugar

Meal Two:

★ 1 Pear

Meal Three:

★ 1 Chicken Breast (grilled) with 1/2 a cup of mixed peppers & 2 lettuce leaves, in a wholemeal wrap
  ★ Add 1 tsp of Homemade Salsa or Mayonnaise
  ★ Glass of Water
★ 1 Cup of Green Tea with Lemon, no added milk or sugar

Meal Four:

★ 1 tbsn of Cottage Cheese on 1 Dark Rye Crisp Bread

Meal Five:

★ 1 Small bowl of Home Made Chilli, using extra lean mince beef
  ★ Glass of Water

Meal Six:

★ 2 tbsp of Natural Greek Yoghurt, a small pinch of Cinnamon and 3-6 Berries

Week Two - Day Two

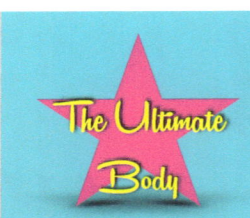

You are nearing the end of Week two and should definitely be feeling amazing by now. You haven't eaten any "processed" goods for nearly two whole weeks and your body will be running on clean and natural energy. What's more, you will certainly have built up the bodies supply of Micronutrients, which will be having incredible effects of the effectiveness of your body and its functions.

Meal One:
★ 2 Egg Omelette, with 1/4 of a cup of Mixed green & Red Peppers & 1/4 of a cup of cooked Ham
  - ★ Glass of Water
  - ★ BCAA
  - ★ MultiVitamin
  - ★ Omega 3, 6 & 9 Capsule
★ 1 Cup of Green Tea & Lemon, no added milk or sugar

Meal Two:
★ 4-5 Unsalted Brazil Nuts

Meal Three:
★ 2 small slices of Smoked Salmon, with Dark Rye Crisp Bread and 1 tbsp of low fat Cream Cheese
  - ★ Glass of Water
★ 1 Cup of Green Tea with Lemon, no added milk or sugar

Meal Four:
★ 1/2 a Banana & 5-8 Berries

Meal Five:
★ 1 Small Baked Potato, served with 1 tin of Tuna and 1 cup of mixed Green Vegetables/Salad
  - ★ Glass of Water

Meal Six:
★ 1 Scoop of Protein Powder mixed with water or Almond Milk

Week Two - Day Six

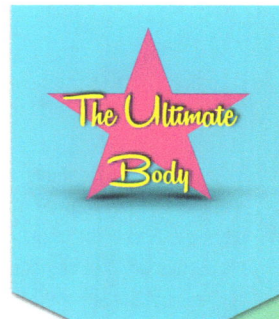

The average human body is made up of between 50 & 65% water, a lot of the human cells require water to exist, including fat cells. By breaking down the cells that are used for energy, we leave toxins and fat floating in the blood stream. When properly hydrated, these toxins are flushed from the system in our urine. That is just one good reason to ensure you are drinking enough water.

Meal One:
★ 1/2 a Cup of Porridge Oats (cooked with water), served with 1/2 a Banana and 6 Berries
  - ★ Glass of Water
  - ★ BCAA
  - ★ MultiVitamin
  - ★ Omega 3, 6 & 9 Capsule
★ 1 Cup of Green Tea & Lemon, no added milk or sugar

Meal Two:
★ 1 Cup of Carrot sticks and 1 tsp of Houmous

Meal Three:
★ 1 Small Lean Grilling Steak, served with 1 cup of mixed Green Vegetables
  - ★ Glass of Water
★ 1 Cup of Green Tea with Lemon, no added milk or sugar

Meal Four:
★ 1/4 of a Cup of Unsalted Almond nuts

Meal Five:
★ 1 Small Fillet of Cod, Served with 1 cup of Steamed mixed Green Vegetables
  - ★ Serve with a squirt of Fresh Lemon Juice (optional)
  - ★ Glass of Water

Meal Six:
★ 2 tbsp of Natural Greek Yoghurt, with 1/2 a scoop of Protein Powder & 2 sliced Strawberries

Week Two - Day Seven

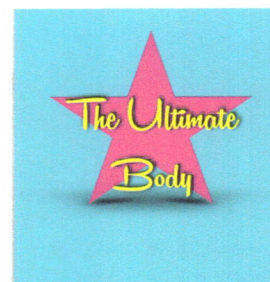

Today is another Treat day, so pick a meal and make it something a little special. Was there something you really fancied earlier in the week? This is your chance to have it. Remember though, portion sizes are still sensible.

It is always worth remembering that you have one treat day per week. It is like a little reward! But remember, if you "fall off the wagon" on another day, then today is no longer a Treat!

Meal One:
★ 1 Egg Fried in Extra Virgin Olive Oil, 2 Small Medallions of Bacon Grilled & fat removed, 2 Stalks of Asparagus
  - ★ Glass of Water
  - ★ BCAA
  - ★ MultiVitamin
  - ★ Omega 3, 6 & 9 Capsule
★ 1 Cup of Green Tea & Lemon, no added milk or sugar

Meal Two:
★ 1/2 a Cup of Unsalted Cashew Nuts

Meal Three:
★ 1/2 a Chicken Breast Sandwich,with Mashed Avocado on 2 Slices of Wholegrain bread
  - ★ You can add 1 tsp of Mayonnaise to the filling
  - ★ Glass of Water
★ 1 Cup of Green Tea with Lemon, no added milk or sugar

Meal Four:
★ 1/2 a Banana

Meal Five:
★ A meal of your choice - Make sure your portions are in moderation
  - ★ Glass of Water

Meal Six:
★ 1/4 Mango, 3 Strawberries & 5 Blueberries, mixed with 1 glass of ice, blended into a smoothie

Week Two

Week Two Review

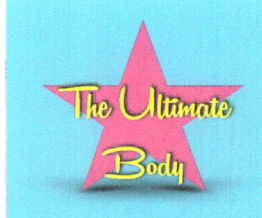

By the end of week two I would expect you are starting to egt use to the routine of eating six times a day. Your body will be a metabolic machine now, churning up all the food regularly and taking all of the nutrients into your bodily systems.

If you weighed yourself before starting, now is the time to step back on to the scales and record your progress.
By now I would expect to see a noticeable change in your size and weight, not to mention how you feel.

Well done, for completing week two!

If you haven't been adding any exercise or activity into your week so far, NOW is the time to get moving. Your results will be boosted along with your energy levels, and believe it or not, Exercise releases the natural feel good hormone (Endorphins), the very same hormone released by Sex and chocolate!

So get moving and start to feel REALLY good in a REALLY healthy way.

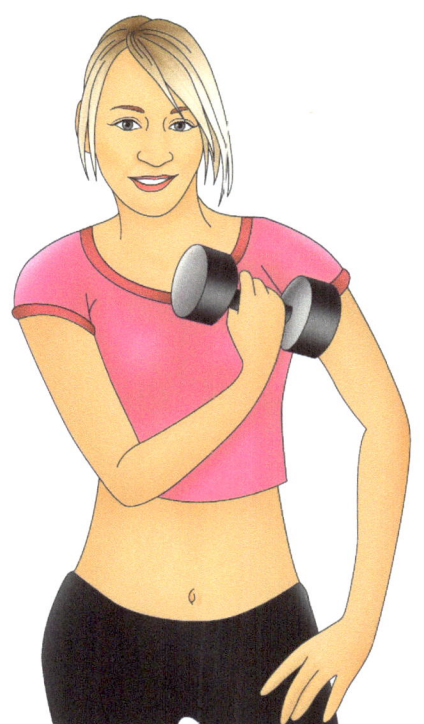

Week Three - Day One

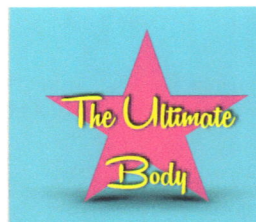

With every day that you successfully stick to the plan, you are building an ever stronger base for your new lifestyle habits. If you can successfully perform one action on a daily basis for 21 days, it becomes a habit, and a healthy habit is never a bad habit.

Meal One:
★ 1/2 a cup of Porridge Oat (cooked in water), with 2 sliced strawberries and 5 blueberries
    ★ Glass of Water
    ★ BCAA
    ★ MultiVitamin
    ★ Omega 3, 6 & 9 Capsule
★ 1 Cup of Green Tea & Lemon, no added milk or sugar

Meal Two:
★ 1 Cup of Celery or Carrot sticks with 1 tsp of Houmous

Meal Three:
★ 1 Tin of Tuna, 2 stalks of Asparagus and 1 cup of mixed Green Vegetables
    ★ Serve with 1 tsp of Mayonnaise
    ★ Glass of Water
★ 1 Cup of Green Tea with Lemon, no added milk or sugar

Meal Four:
★ 1/2 a cup of mixed unsalted nuts (cashew, brazil, macadamia, money nuts, almonds)

Meal Five:
★ 1 Salmon Fillet, 1 cup of Rocket, 1/2 a Cup of Kale, 1/2 a Cup of chopped Carrots, 1/2 a cup of Broccoli
    ★ Glass of Water

Meal Six:
★ 2 tbsp of Natural Greek Yoghurt, with 1 small pinch of Cinnamon & 1/2 a banana sliced

If you are not already being active, try and do 30-60 minutes of exercise today. You can either follow the Ultimate Body 12 week Workout, join a gym or fitness class or go for a nice walk in the sunshine.

Week Three - Day Two

You may have already seen some progress with your shape and weight loss, but adding activity into your weekly plan now is going to amplify those results.

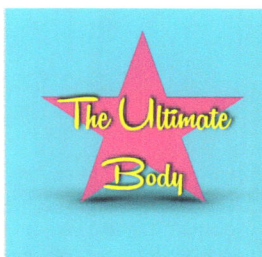

Meal One:

★ 2 Eggs boiled & Sliced, on 1 slice of Rye Bread Toasted
- ★ Glass of Water
- ★ BCAA
- ★ MultiVitamin
- ★ Omega 3, 6 & 9 Capsule

★ 1 Cup of Green Tea & Lemon, no added milk or sugar

Meal Two:

★ 1 Pear

Meal Three:

★ 1 Grilled Chicken Breast, Sliced with Mixed red & green peppers, 1 lettuce leaf, in a wholemeal Wrap
- ★ Serve with 1 tsp of Mayonnaise or Home made Salsa
- ★ Glass of Water

★ 1 Cup of Green Tea with Lemon, no added milk or sugar

Meal Four:

★ 1 Scoop of Protein powder mixed with water or almond milk

Meal Five:

★ 1 Grilled Pork Chop, served with 1 cup of mixed green Vegetables & 1/2 and avocado sliced
- ★ Glass of Water

Meal Six:

★ 1/2 a cup of mixed Berries

Week Three - Day Three

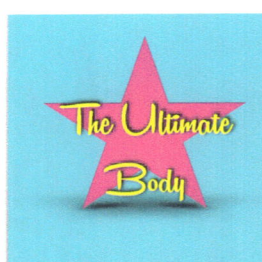

Now you should be starting to recognise healthy foods and unhealthy foods with ease, you probably will not have much fancy for stodgy, heavy meals. As you start to adapt, you can start to change a few ingredients around for your meal options. Picking something similar but different, can make a big difference in your enjoyment of your food.... and food should be enjoyed!

Meal One:

★ 3 Strawberries, 1/3 Mango, 1/2 Banana & 1 glass of ice, mixed in a blender until Smooth
    ★ BCAA
    ★ MultiVitamin
    ★ Omega 3, 6 & 9 Capsule
★ 1 Cup of Green Tea & Lemon, no added milk or sugar

Meal Two:

★ 1 Tbsp of Cottage Cheese on 1 Dark Rye Crisp Bread

Meal Three:

★ 1/2 a Turkey Breast Grilled, served with 1/2 a cup of cucumber, 2 cherry tomatoes and 3 asparagus stalks
    ★ Serve with 1 tsp of Mayonnaise or Home made Salsa
    ★ Glass of Water
★ 1 Cup of Green Tea with Lemon, no added milk or sugar

Meal Four:

★ 1 cup of unsalted Almond nuts

Meal Five:

★ 1 loin of Swordfish Grilled, served with 2 cups of mixed leaf salad
    ★ Glass of Water

Meal Six:

★ 1 tbsp of Natural Greek Yoghurt, 1 Scoop of Protein Powder, 1 small pinch of Cinnamon

Today you should try and get in some more activity. It doesn't have to be the same as Day one, but 30-60 minutes of movement will boost your weight loss results.

Week Three - Day Four

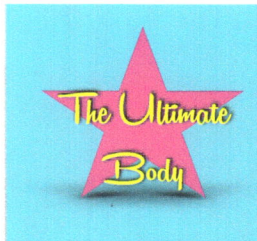

Portion control should no longer be an issue for you, your stomach will be well adapted to the size and frequency of the meals you have been having and will have started to shrink to a size more fitting of this. Making you feel fuller for longer and satisfied with how much you are consuming on a daily basis.

Meal One:
★ 2 Sardines (in water) on 1 slice of Rye Bread Toasted
  ★ BCAA
  ★ MultiVitamin
  ★ Omega 3, 6 & 9 Capsule
★ 1 Cup of Green Tea & Lemon, no added milk or sugar

Meal Two:
★ 4 Cherry Tomatoes

Meal Three:
★ 1 Small Baked Potato, with a 1/3 of a cup of grated cheese (add NO butter)
  ★ Glass of Water
★ 1 Cup of Green Tea with Lemon, no added milk or sugar

Meal Four:
★ 1/2 a Banana

Meal Five:
★ 1 Bowl of Home Made Vegetable Soup, served with 2 slices of Rye Bread
  ★ Glass of Water

Meal Six:
★ 1/2 a cup of mixed berries

Week Three - Day Five

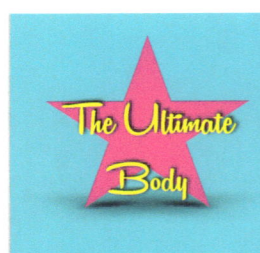

You should always keep in mind that what you are doing is not a diet with an expiration date, it is a lifestyle alteration that will lead to a healthier & slimmer body. Once this Four week Meal Plan Guide is completed, you should have enough knowledge and will have built up enough good habits, that you can continue to eat similar meals that you have created yourself.

Meal One:
★ Porridge Oats (cooked in Water) Served with a small pinch of Cinnamon and 1/2 a cup of mixed fruits
  ★ BCAA
  ★ MultiVitamin
  ★ Omega 3, 6 & 9 Capsule
★ 1 Cup of Green Tea & Lemon, no added milk or sugar

Meal Two:
★ 1 Cup of Carrot sticks with Mayonnaise or Houmous

Meal Three:
★ 1 Grilled Chicken Breast, served with 1 cup of mixed Green Vegetables & 2 Asparagus Stalks
  ★ Glass of Water
★ 1 Cup of Green Tea with Lemon, no added milk or sugar

Meal Four:
★ 1/2 a cup of mixed unsalted nuts

Meal Five:
★ 1 Bowl of Home Made Chilli Con Carne
  ★ Glass of Water

Meal Six:
★ 2 tbsp of Natural Greek Yoghurt with 6 berries

Today would be another great day to incorporate some activity into your week, another 30-60 minutes would be ideal.

Week Three

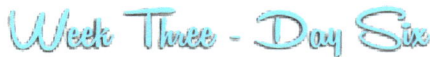

Week Three - Day Six

Your actions will create a reaction in your body, your results should, by now be visible and when looking in the mirror you will be seeing changes to your shape and figure.

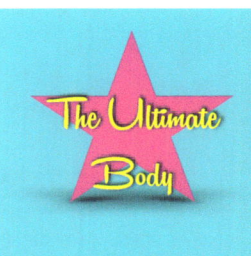

Meal One:
- ★ 1/2 a Banana, 5 Raspberries and 8 Blueberries, with 1 glass of ice, blended until smooth
    - ★ BCAA
    - ★ MultiVitamin
    - ★ Omega 3, 6 & 9 Capsule
- ★ 1 Cup of Green Tea & Lemon, no added milk or sugar

Meal Two:
- ★ 1 scoop of protein Powder mixed with water or Almond Milk

Meal Three:
- ★ 1 Smoked Mackerel Fillet, served with 1 cup of mixed vegetables
    - ★ Glass of Water
- ★ 1 Cup of Green Tea with Lemon, no added milk or sugar

Meal Four:
- ★ 1 cup of Carrot stick with 1 tsp of houmous or Mayonnaise

Meal Five:
- ★ 2 cups of Extra Lean Mince Beef, with Home Made Tomato Sauce, served with a small handful of wholemeal Pasta
    - ★ Glass of Water

Meal Six:
- ★ 1/2 a cup of mixed unsalted nuts

Week Three - Day Seven

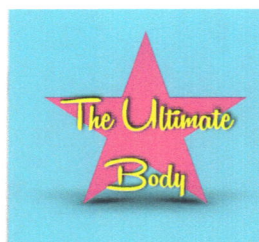

You have successfully made it to your third Treat day! Well done. By now you will know that treat day means one meal can be a little naughty, as reward if you like. portions are still in moderation, but it is a big treat!

Meal One:

★ 2 Egg Omelette, made with 1/2 a cup of mixed peppers and 1/4 of a cup of grated cheese.
  - ★ BCAA
  - ★ MultiVitamin
  - ★ Omega 3, 6 & 9 Capsule
★ 1 Cup of Green Tea & Lemon, no added milk or sugar

Meal Two:

★ 1 Apple or Pear

Meal Three:

★ 1 Grilled Chicken Breast, served with 2 cups of Mixed salad & 1 tsp of Houmous or Mayonnaise
  - ★ Glass of Water
★ 1 Cup of Green Tea with Lemon, no added milk or sugar

Meal Four:

★ 1/3 of a cup of mixed unsalted nuts

Meal Five:

★ A meal of your choice, portions sizes should be controlled
  - ★ Glass of Water

Meal Six:

★ 2 tbsp of Natural Greek Yoghurt, with 1 small pinch of grated Dark Chocolate (80% cocoa of greater)

Week Three Review

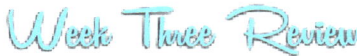

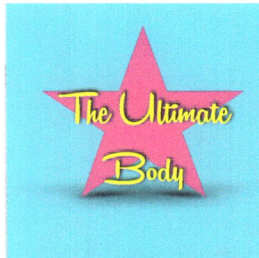

That's another week passed, and if you have stuck to the plan for all of this time, your habits should be really starting to change now as we pass the 21 day mark.

I know that you are probably itching to step on the bathroom scales, but refrain from doing this until the end of next week.

If you are attending fitness classes or the gym, try and do some resistance training, using either weights or your own body weight. If you are in a gym, ask a member of staff to help you with which machines and exercises to do.

For now, well done and enjoy your fourth and final week of following The Ultimate Body L.E.A.N. Guide plan.

Week Four - Day One

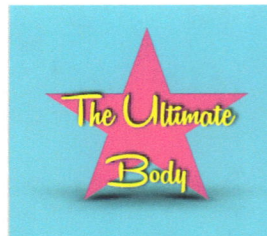

It's time for you to start making decisions now. So for your main dinner meal, or meal number 5 of every day this week, you will pick your own choices, either meals you have enjoyed from the plan or you can start to manage your own meals. Use your cup for portion control. I know you are going to be absolutely

Have you looked in the mirror recently? Are you starting to see the changes? How have you been feeling? Are your energy levels UP? Is exercise not as bad as you thought it might be?

Your health is improving! Keep going!

Meal One:
★ 1/2 a cup of Porridge oats (cooked with Water), serve with 1/2 a cup of mixed fruits
  ★ BCAA
  ★ MultiVitamin
  ★ Omega 3, 6 & 9 Capsule
★ 1 Cup of Green Tea & Lemon, no added milk or sugar

Meal Two:
★ 1/2 cup of raw Green Beans

Meal Three:
★ 1 Grilled Chicken Breast, Sliced with Mixed red & green peppers, 1 lettuce leaf, in a wholemeal Wrap
  ★ Glass of Water
★ 1 Cup of Green Tea with Lemon, no added milk or sugar

Meal Four:
★ 1/2 a Banana

Meal Five:
★ A meal of your choice, portions sizes should be controlled
  ★ Glass of Water

Meal Six:
★ 1/2 a cup of unsalted Macadamia Nuts

Week Four - Day Two

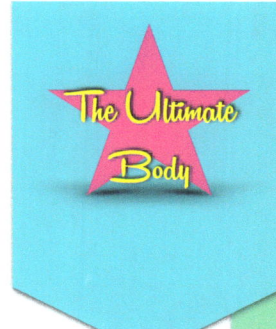

Meal One:
★ 2 Egg Omelette, made with 1/2 a cup of mixed peppers and 1/4 of a cup of grated cheese.
  ★ BCAA
  ★ MultiVitamin
  ★ Omega 3, 6 & 9 Capsule
★ 1 Cup of Green Tea & Lemon, no added milk or sugar

Meal Two:
★ 2 tbsp of Natural Greek Yoghurt & 6-10 Blueberries

Meal Three:
★ 1 Smoked Mackerel Fillet, served with 1 cup of mixed vegetables
  ★ Glass of Water
★ 1 Cup of Green Tea with Lemon, no added milk or sugar

Meal Four:
★ 1 cup of celery or carrot sticks with 1 tsp of houmous or Mayonnaise

Meal Five:
★ A meal of your choice, portions sizes should be controlled
  ★ Glass of Water

Meal Six:
★ 1/2 a banana

Week Four - Day Three

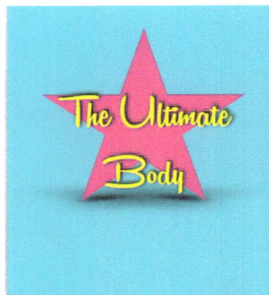

Meal One:
★ 2 Scrambled Eggs on 1 Slices of Rye Bread Toasted
    ★ BCAA
    ★ MultiVitamin
    ★ Omega 3, 6 & 9 Capsule
★ 1 Cup of Green Tea & Lemon, no added milk or sugar

Meal Two:
★ 1 Apple or Pear

Meal Three:
★ 1 Tin of Salmon, mixed with 1 tbsp of Mayonnaise, served with 2 Dark Rye Crispbreads
    ★ Glass of Water
★ 1 Cup of Green Tea with Lemon, no added milk or sugar

Meal Four:
★ 1/3 of a cup of unsalted Almond nuts

Meal Five:
★ A meal of your choice, portions sizes should be controlled
    ★ Glass of Water

Meal Six:
★ 6-10 Berries

Week Four - Day Four

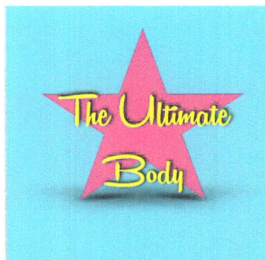

Meal One:

★ 2 Sardines (in Water) on 1 Slice of Rye Bread Toasted
   ★ BCAA
   ★ MultiVitamin
   ★ Omega 3, 6 & 9 Capsule
★ 1 Cup of Green Tea & Lemon, no added milk or sugar

Meal Two:

★ 1 tbsp of Cottage Cheese on 1 Dark Rye Crispbread

Meal Three:

★ 1 Grilled Chicken Breast, served with 1/2 cup of mixed peppers, served in a Wholemeal Wrap
   ★ Add a tsp of Mayonnaise (optional)
   ★ Glass of Water
★ 1 Cup of Green Tea with Lemon, no added milk or sugar

Meal Four:

★ 1 Apple

Meal Five:

★ A meal of your choice, portions sizes should be controlled
   ★ Glass of Water

Meal Six:

★ 1 Scoop of Protein Powder mixed with water or Almond Milk

Week Four - Day Five

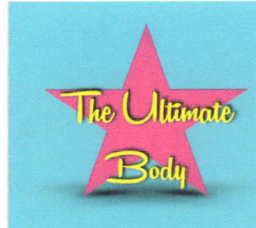

Meal One:
★ 1/4 Mango, 6 Blueberries and 1/2 a Banana, mixed with 1 class of ice in a blender until smooth

- ★ BCAA
- ★ MultiVitamin
- ★ Omega 3, 6 & 9 Capsule

★ 1 Cup of Green Tea & Lemon, no added milk or sugar

Meal Two:
★ 1/2 a cup of Carrot sticks with 1 tsp of Houmous

Meal Three:
★ 1 Tin of Tuna (in water) with 2 Asparagus Stalks and 1/2 a cup of Mixed Green Vegetables
- ★ Glass of Water

★ 1 Cup of Green Tea with Lemon, no added milk or sugar

Meal Four:
★ 2 tbsp of Organic Peanut Butter

Meal Five:
★ A meal of your choice, portions sizes should be controlled
- ★ Glass of Water

Meal Six:
★ 1/2 a cup of mixed unsalted nuts

Week Four - Day Six

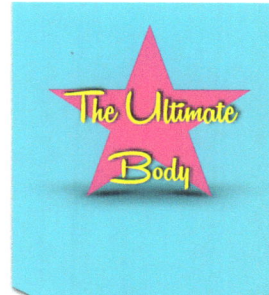

Meal One:

★ 1/2 a cup of Porridge oats (cooked in water), serve with 6-8 blueberries and 1/2 a banana
  - ★ BCAA
  - ★ MultiVitamin
  - ★ Omega 3, 6 & 9 Capsule

★ 1 Cup of Green Tea & Lemon, no added milk or sugar

Meal Two:

★ 2 boiled eggs sliced

Meal Three:

★ Home Made Vegetable Soup
  - ★ Glass of Water

★ 1 Cup of Green Tea with Lemon, no added milk or sugar

Meal Four:

★ 1 Apple or Pear

Meal Five:

★ A meal of your choice, portions sizes should be controlled
  - ★ Glass of Water

Meal Six:

★ 1/4 of a cup of unsalted brazil buts

Week Four - Day Seven

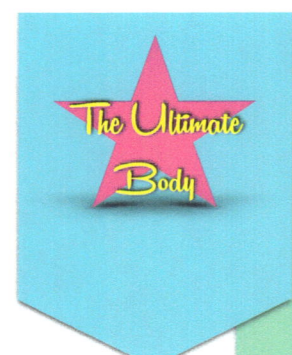

Meal One:

★ 2 Sardines (in water) on 1 slice of Sunflower Rye Bread (toasted)
  ★ BCAA
  ★ MultiVitamin
  ★ Omega 3, 6 & 9 Capsule
★ 1 Cup of Green Tea & Lemon, no added milk or sugar

Meal Two:

★ 1 scoop of Protein Powder mixed with water or almond milk

Meal Three:

★ 2 slices of smoked Salmon with wholegrain Crispbreads, serve with houmous or mayonnaise
  ★ Glass of Water
★ 1 Cup of Green Tea with Lemon, no added milk or sugar

Meal Four:

★ 1 tbsp of Cottage Cheese on 1 Dark Rye Crispbread

Meal Five:

★ A meal of your choice, portions sizes should be controlled
  ★ Glass of Water

Meal Six:

★ 2 tbsp of Natural Greek Yoghurt, with 1 small pinch of grated Dark Chocolate (80% cocoa of greater)

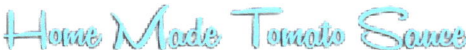 Home Made Tomato Sauce

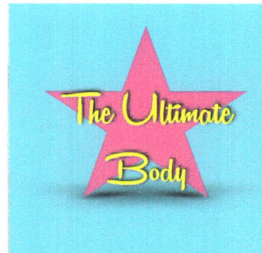

That is it, you have completed the Four weeks of the Ultimate Body Meal Plan. Now you should have enough knowledge of the foods you have been eating and what is healthy and what isn't to make your own choices.

But don't worry, you can continue to follow the meals in this plan if you want to and if you have enjoyed them.

But now for something important! It is now time to take your weight on the scales AND a progress photo to look at against the original first photo. You should take these photos every 4 weeks to monitor your physical changes, but you should also remember to take note of your psychological changes as well, like how you have been feeling.

Eating a healthy diet isn't just about weight control, it is about being HEALTHY!

Let me know how you have got on on the plan, as I love to hear peoples progress stories.
You can always get in touch with me as well, by emailing lesley@lmfitness.info
Why not send me your progress photos? I'd love to see them!

You can also Tweet me @LmFitness or Instagram me @LMFITNESS1

I hope you have achieved what you wanted to with this meal plan, and don't give up now... Keep Going!

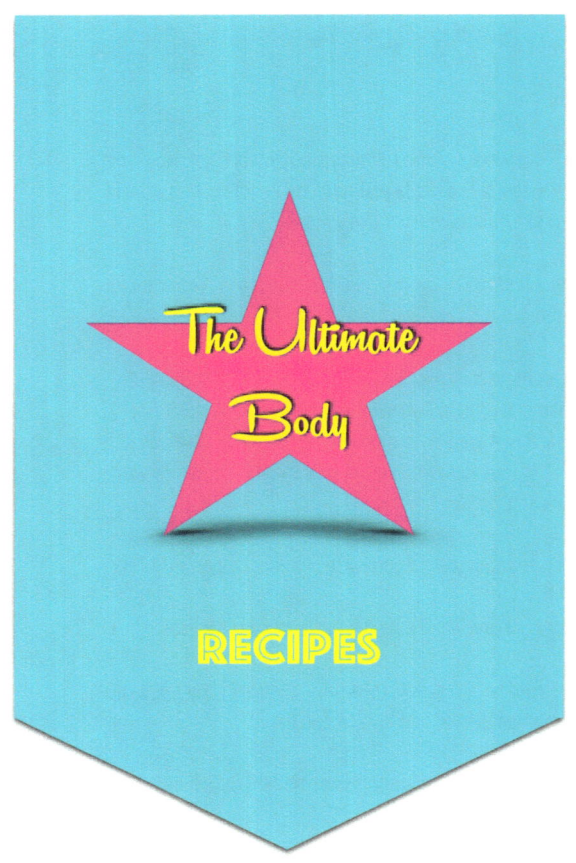

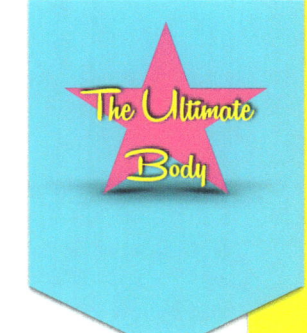

Ingredients for 4 Servings

- ★ Low calorie cooking spray
- ★ 2 shallots, finely chopped
- ★ 2 garlic cloves, crushed
- ★ 225g button mushrooms, thinly sliced
- ★ 1 x 400g can chopped tomatoes
- ★ Salt and freshly ground black pepper

Instructions:

- ★ Spray a pan with low calorie cooking spray and cook the shallots and garlic for 2–3 minutes until just softened.
- ★ Stir in the mushrooms and cook for 1 minute. Add the chopped tomatoes.
- ★ Reduce the heat and simmer for about 15 minutes until reduced and thickened. Check the seasoning.
- ★ Add some Oregano or Mixed Herbs for added Flavour.
- ★ Add the Cooked Extra Lean Mince to the mixture and allow to reduce for a further few minutes.

Home Made Salsa

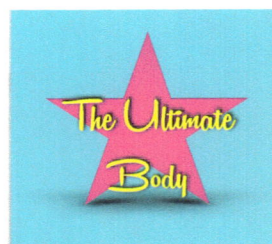

Ingredients for 12-15 servings:

- ★ 3 large ripe tomatoes, diced or 1 (14-ounce) can diced tomatoes with their juice
- ★ 1 small onion, finely chopped
- ★ 1 small green bell pepper, seeds and veins removed, and minced
- ★ 1 (4-ounce) can chopped green chiles with juice
- ★ 1 clove garlic, minced
- ★ 1 tablespoon olive oil

Instructions:

Combine all ingredients, and any extra ingredients you may want to add, in a large bowl. Stir well with a spoon. Cover with plastic wrap and chill until serving time.

Home Made Chilli Con Carne

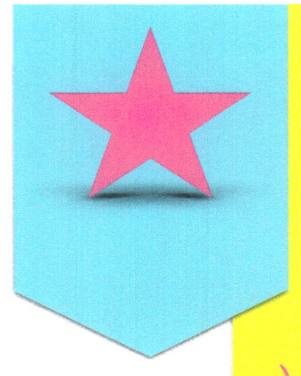

Ingredients:

- 1 tbsp oil
- 1 large onion
- 1 red pepper
- 2 garlic cloves, peeled
- 1 heaped tsp hot chilli powder (or 1 level tbsp if you only have mild)
- 1 tsp paprika
- 1 tsp ground cumin
- 500g lean minced beef
- 400g can chopped tomatoes
- ½ tsp dried marjoram
- 410g can red kidney beans

Instructions:

Prepare the vegetables. Chop The onion into small dice. Cut 1 red pepper in half lengthways, remove stalk and wash the seeds away, then chop. Peel and finely chop the garlic.

Put your pan on the hob over a medium heat. Add the oil and leave it for 1-2 minutes until hot. Add the onions and cook, stirring frequently, until the onions are soft. Add the garlic, red pepper, 1 level tbsp mild chilli powder, 1 tsp paprika and 1 tsp ground cumin. Give it all a stir, and leave to cook for 5 minutes, stirring occasionally.

Brown 500g lean minced beef. Add your meat to the vegetables. Keep stirring and prodding, until all the mince is in mixed in and fully cooked.

Add 1 can of chopped tomatoes (400g can). Tip in ½ tsp dried marjoram, and add a good pinch of salt and pepper.

Bring the whole thing to the boil, give it a good stir and put a lid on the pan. Turn down the heat until it is gently simmering and leave it for about 20 minutes. You stir occasionally After simmering gently, the saucy mince mixture should look thick and juicy.

Drain and rinse 1 can of red kidney beans (410g can) in a sieve and stir them into the chilli pot. Bring to the boil again, and gently simmer without the lid for another 10 minutes, adding a little more water if it looks too dry. Taste for season. Replace the lid, turn off the heat and leave to stand for 10 minutes before serving.

Home Made Vegetable Soup

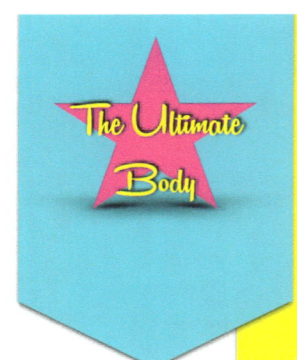

The Ultimate Body

Combine baby carrots, potatoes, onion, celery, beans, cabbage, tomatoes, green beans, chicken broth, **vegetable** stock, water, basil, sage, thyme, and salt in a large pot; bring to a boil. Reduce heat to low; cover. Simmer until **vegetables** are tender, about 90 minutes.

You can pick and choose your vegetables, however this is how I always make vegetable soup.

Recipes

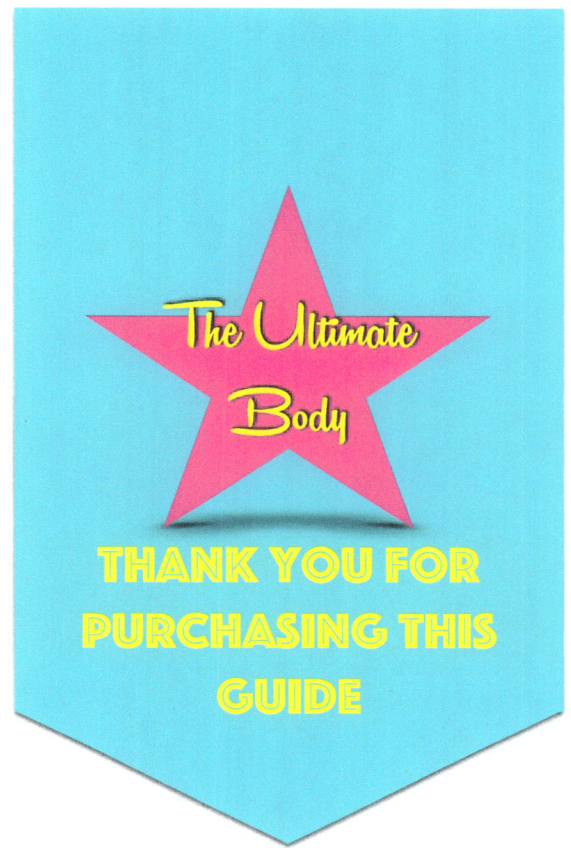

I wish you EVERY success with your health & fitness journey, whatever your goal is. Remember to send me your progress photos and let me know how you get on with the meal plans.

Twitter: @LmFitness
Instagram: @LMFITNESS1
Email: lesley@lmfitness.info

www.ingramcontent.com/pod-product-compliance
Lightning Source LLC
Chambersburg PA
CBHW060835290526
45792CB00006BB/1937